NATURAL DIABETES TREATMENT

DR MIRIAM KINAI

ISBN: 1490488995

ISBN-13: 978-1490488998

CONTENTS

ACKNOWLEDGMENTS

I would like to express my sincere gratitude to everyone who contributed in one way or another to the development of this publication.

I would especially like to thank http://www.zazzle.com/ChristianArtGifts for their photographs.

1

DIET THERAPY

The diabetic diet is a very important aspect of natural diabetes treatment since diabetic foods can aid blood sugar regulation. Dietary modifications that you can institute to complement your conventional diabetes mellitus treatment include:

1.

Eat a high fiber breakfast

Begin your day by eating a high fiber breakfast cereal since it is an excellent source of water soluble fiber which reduces the rate at which carbohydrates are absorbed and thus maintains steadier blood sugar levels. In addition, increase the benefits of your breakfast by adding a cup of chopped fruit to your cereal.

***

2.

Eat more beans

Increase your intake of beans since they are rich in water soluble fiber which reduces the rate at which the blood glucose rises after meals and this helps with the stabilization of blood glucose levels throughout the day. In addition, beans are also filling and thus valuable when trying to limit caloric intake.

3.

Eat more vegetables

Increase your intake of vegetables to 5 servings each day as they are rich in nutrients and fiber which reduces the rapid rise in blood sugar levels after a meal. Vegetables are also filing, low in fat and calories and thus help in loosing excess body weight. Note that 1 vegetable serving is I cup of raw vegetables or ½ cup of cooked vegetables.

4.

Eat more magnesium rich foods

Increase the intake of magnesium as it may help achieve better blood sugar control by eating ample green leafy vegetables such as spinach as well as whole grains, beans, and broccoli every day.

5.

Eat more chromium rich foods

Increase your chromium intake since it is useful for blood sugar regulation by eating more cheese, meat and brown rice.

***

6.

Eat or drink more cinnamon

Increase you intake of cinnamon as it may help you lower blood sugar level by steeping cinnamon sticks in hot water to brew cinnamon tea or by sprinkling powdered cinnamon on your yoghurt, whole grain toast, baked fish, and chicken dishes.

***

7.

Eat more nuts

Go nuts and increase your intake of nuts as these are rich in fiber, magnesium as well as antioxidants and thus may help prevent diabetic eye and nerve complications.

***

8.

Avoid simple sugars

Avoid simple sugars like sucrose from table sugar and fructose from fruit juices because they cause the blood sugar to rise and fall rapidly.

***

9.

Avoid refined grains

Avoid refined grains such as white bread, pasta, and rice and replace them with whole grains such as brown bread, pasta, and rice to stabilize blood sugar levels and provide more nutrients and fiber.

***

10.

Avoid high glycemic index foods

Avoid foods with high glycemic indexes like processed white flour cakes or doughnuts and eat more low glycemic index foods.

Foods with a glycemic index of less than 20 include:

Peanuts, Broccoli, Cucumber, Lettuce, Spinach, Tomatoes, Green beans, Low fat yogurt

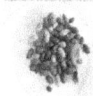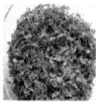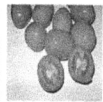

Foods with a glycemic index of 20- 30 include:

Whole milk, Soya milk, Cherries

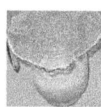

Foods with a glycemic index of 30- 40 include:

Whole wheat spaghetti, Skimmed milk, Apples, Pears

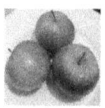

Foods with a glycemic index of 40-50 include:

All bran cereal, Multi grain bread, Apple juice, Carrot juice, Pineapple juice, Oranges

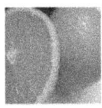

Foods with glycemic index of 50- 60 include:

Bananas, Mangoes, Sweet potatoes, Boiled potatoes, Oat bran, Brown rice, Popcorn, Orange juice

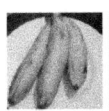 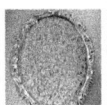 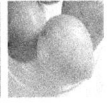

Foods with a glycemic index of 60- 70 include:

Whole meal bread

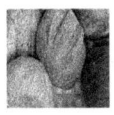

*, *, *, *, *

2

SUPPLEMENTS

Nutritional supplements that can help lower high blood sugar include:

1.

Alpha-lipoic acid

Alpha-lipoic acid, which is also known as ALA, lipoic acid and thiotic acid, is an antioxidant. This means that it reduces free radical damage which causes nerve damage and other complications in the body. ALA is therefore used to ease the nerve pains, numbness, tingling, and burning sensations associated with diabetic nerve complications. Though ALA, which is usually given at doses of 600 to 800 milligrams a day, can also lower blood sugar levels, more research is needed to determine its true role in the management of diabetes. It is naturally found in spinach, broccoli, liver, and potatoes.

***

2.

Chromium

Though chromium supplements, which are usually given at doses of 200 micrograms daily, can lower blood sugar levels, more research is needed to determine their true role in the management of diabetes. Good dietary sources of this essential trace mineral include whole grains and meat.

3.

Omega 3 fatty acids

Omega 3 fatty acids can benefit diabetic patients with heart disease since studies have shown that they can lower the levels of triglycerides. Good dietary sources of omega 3 fatty acids include oily fish, fish oil, wheat germ, canola oil, soya bean oil, and walnuts.

4.

A daily multi-vitamin

Take a daily multi-vitamin and multi-mineral supplement that is well balanced and that contains:

a) Magnesium as it may help achieve better blood sugar control.

b) The B vitamins as these are vital especially for those who have developed neuropathies or diabetic nerve complications.

c) Vitamins A, C, and E and the mineral selenium as these antioxidants may help reduce the free radical damage to various organs in the body.

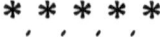

3

HERBS

Herbs that are used to manage diabetes include:

1.

Cinnamon

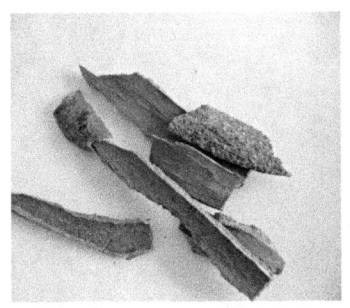 A German study proved that cinnamon improves blood sugar control in people with type 2 diabetes by reducing their blood glucose level. This can be achieved by taking just 1/2 teaspoon of cinnamon each day.

Cinnamon can also prevent diabetes. This was shown by a study done by *The Center for Applied Health Sciences* in which participants who were given 250mg of water soluble cinnamon each day were found to have an increase in the antioxidants associated with lowering blood glucose levels.

***

2.

Fenugreek

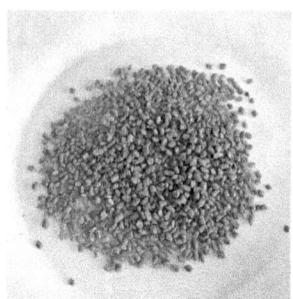

A study published in the European Journal of Clinical Nutrition found that patients with type 1 diabetes who took 50 grams of fenugreek (Trigonella foenum-graecum) seed powder twice a day had lower blood glucose levels than those who did not. In addition to lowering blood glucose levels, these seeds which are used in Indian cooking, are also thought to reduce high cholesterol levels.

***

3.

American Ginseng

A study found that patients with type 2 diabetes who took 3 grams of American ginseng each day had lower fasting blood sugar levels and lower glycosylated hemoglobin levels than those who didn't. In addition to its blood sugar lowering capabilities, ginseng is also known for its immune boosting effects.

***

4.

Garlic

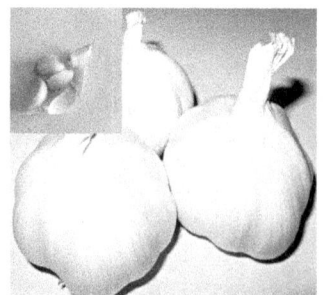

Garlic is also thought to lower blood sugar levels though more research is required.

***

Other herbs that are said to be useful in the management of diabetes include:

1. Aloe (Aloe vera)

2. Asian ginseng (Panax quinquefolius)

3. Bitter melon (Momordica charantia)

4. Gurmar (Gymnema sylvestre)

5. Prickly-pear cactus (Opuntia spp)

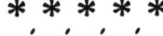

4

ESSENTIAL OILS

Aromatherapy is the use of essential oils for their healing benefits.

Though aromatherapy has not been proven to cure diabetes, essential oils can be used to help treat complications of diabetes like skin infections and chronic stress.

Essential oils that are used to manage diabetes include relaxing lavender essential oil and antiseptic tea tree essential oil.

Lavender Essential Oil

Botanical name: Lavendula officinalis

Perfumery Note: Middle note

Lavender Essential Oil Safety Information

1. Do not use it in pregnancy especially the first 3 months.

2. Do not use it if you are breastfeeding.

3. Do not use it on young children as it may cause breast development in boys (gynaecomastia) and girls (pre-pubescent breast development).

4. Avoid it if you have low blood pressure as you may feel drowsy after using it.

***

Tea Tree Essential Oil

Botanical Name: Melaleuca alternifolia

Perfumery Note: Top note

Tea Tree Essential Oil Safety Information

1. It may be irritating on sensitive skins.

2. It may cause sweating when used in high concentrations. Maximum recommended level is 0.1%.

***

Using Essential Oils for Diabetes Treatment

The first step in using essential oils to manage diabetes is to do a patch test for each of the essential oils that you want to use.

To do this, simply apply the essential oil that has been diluted with a carrier oil on the inner aspect of your elbow, bandage it and wait for 24 hours to see if you will develop rashes or swelling or any other sign of an allergic reaction. If you do, do not use that essential oil.

Foot Bath. Create your own antiseptic foot bath by adding 3 drops of lavender and 3 drops of tea tree essential oils to a bowl of warm water. If you have decreased sensation due to diabetic nerve complications, ask someone to check the temperature of the footbath for you.

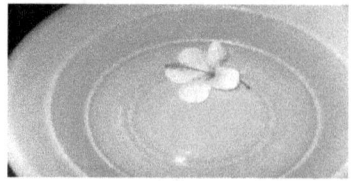

Antiseptic Wash. Add 10 drops of lavender essential oil and 15 drops of tea tree essential oil to ½ cup (4 oz or 125 ml) of warm water, dip cotton balls in it and use it to cleanse diabetic ulcers.

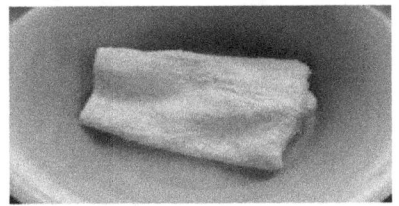

Antiseptic Dressing. Add 1 drop of lavender essential oil and 2 drops of tea tree essential oil to 5 ml of sweet almond oil. Put a few drops of this mixture on a gauze and use it to dress a diabetic ulcer as it may aid its healing.

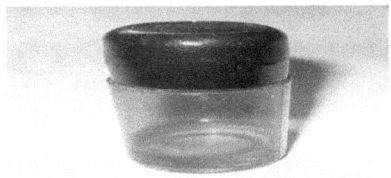

Body Massage Oil. Add 50 drops (2.5 ml) of lavender essential oil to one cup (8oz or 250 ml) of sweet almond oil or sunflower oil or any other carrier oil to create a body massage oil. Get a massage from a professional massage therapist or a loved one at least once a month.

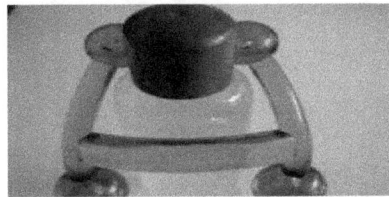

Aloe Vera Aromatherapy Gel. Add 50 drops of lavender essential oil to one cup (8 oz or 250 ml) of natural aloe vera gel to create a non-greasy, healing moisturizer.

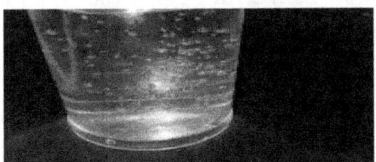

Bath Gel. Add 50 drops (2.5 ml or ½ teaspoons) of relaxing lavender essential oil to one cup (8 oz or 250 ml) of unscented bath gel or liquid soap to create a relaxing bath gel.

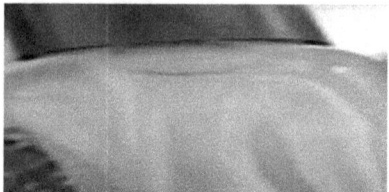

Bath Salts. Mix 2 cups of Epsom salts, 1 cup of sea salt and 1 cup of baking soda. Add 50 drops (2.5 ml or ½ teaspoons) of lavender essential oil and a few drops of food coloring (optional) to create your own bath salts. Add one cup to your bath water for a relaxing soak.

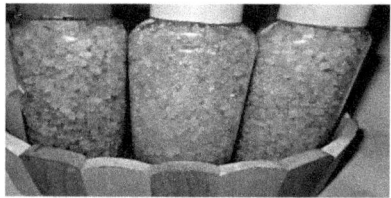

Hand and Foot Oil. Add 2 drops lavender essential oil and 2 drops of tea tree essential oil to 20 ml of a carrier oil like sweet almond oil. Use it to massage your feet after your foot bath before you wrap them in soft cotton socks. You can also use it to massage your hands.

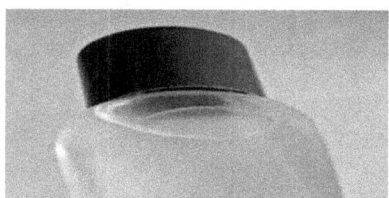

Beeswax Hand cream. Melt 4 tablespoons of beeswax tablespoons and 2 tablespoons of shea butter. Remove from the heat source and add 8 tablespoons of sweet almond oil or any other carrier oil you may have. Mix thoroughly and then add 10 drops of lavender essential oil.

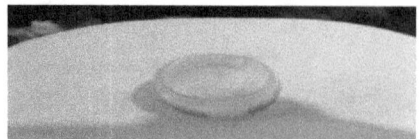

Aromatherapy Bath. Create a relaxing bath by dispersing 12 drops of lavender essential oils in your warm bath water. You can also mix it with milk to help it disperse.

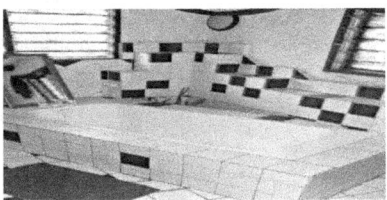

Inhalation Balls.

Add 6 drops of relaxing lavender essential oil to your handkerchief or a cotton ball or sponge and sniff it throughout the day whenever you begin to feel tense.

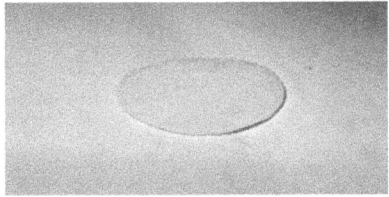

Body Lotion

Heat 6 oz or 190 ml of sweet almond oil and 1.5 oz or 45 grams of grated beeswax in a double boiler or water bath until the beeswax melts and mixes completely with the vegetable oils. Remove the mixture from the heat and let it cool completely. Put 8 oz or 250 ml water in a blender and with the blender on high speed, slowly pour in the cooled vegetable oil and beeswax mixture. Blend until the mixture emulsifies and forms a thick, creamy lotion. Add 10-20 drops of lavender essential oil drop by drop as you blend until you get your required scent. Pour your lotion in a glass jar.

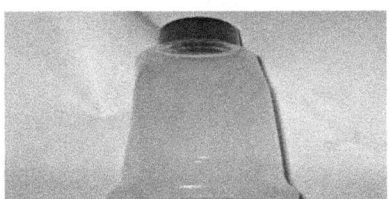

Personal Perfume.

Put 10 ml jojoba in a bottle and add 60 drops of lavender essential oil followed by 10 ml of 99% alcohol isopropyl in a spray bottle to make your own relaxing perfume.

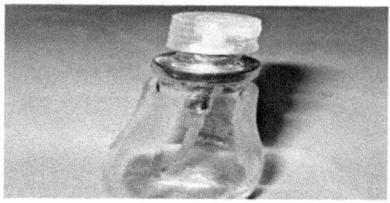

Room Fragrance.

Add 24 drops of lavender essential oil to your diffuser. If your diffuser comes with instructions, use the number of drops recommended by the manufacturer.

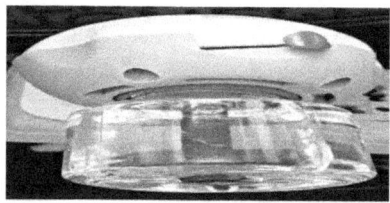

Room Scent.

Add 12 drops of lavender essential oil to ¼ cup (2 oz or 60 ml) of water, place it on an oil warmer and light the candle to disperse the relaxing and healing scent.

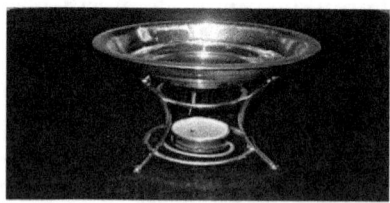

Light Bulb Scent.

Drop 3 drops of lavender essential oil to a light bulb when the light is switched off, switch it on to illuminate and scent your room.

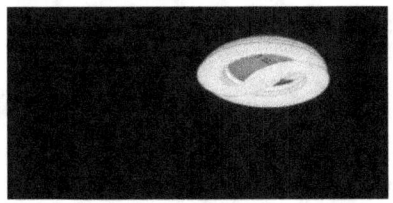

Aroma Ring Scent.

Add 5 drops of lavender essential oil to an aroma oil ring, place it on top of your lamp bulb, light the lamp and experience therapeutic lighting.

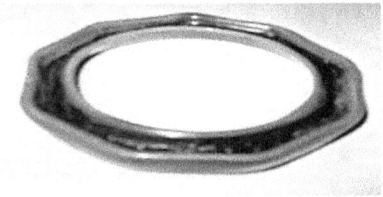

Car Diffuser.

Add lavender essential oil to your car's diffuser according to the manufacturer's instructions and let the healing scent envelope you as you drive.

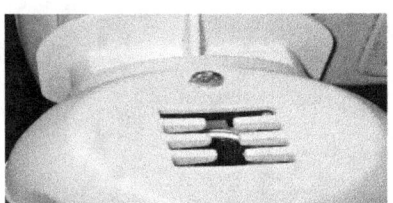

* * * * *

5

LIFESTYLE MODIFICATIONS

Lifestyle modifications that can help manage diabetes include:

1.

Regular Exercise

Regular exercise is very important for regulating blood sugar since it aids:

a. Loosing excess weight

b. Regulating blood sugar levels especially for overweight and obese diabetics

c. Regular aerobic exercise also reduces the amount of insulin needed

d. Weight bearing exercises increases muscle mass, improves metabolic efficiency and strengthen muscles, tendons and ligaments.

Therefore begin exercising regularly but if you have been leading a sedentary lifestyle, consult your doctor and nutritionist before making changes to your exercise regimen. When you do begin exercising, train under the supervision of a qualified person especially if you have developed diabetic eye complications.

In addition, invest in a good pair of sports shoes that will cushion your feet and redistribute your weight evenly as you walk, jog, jump or run. If you develop calluses, consult a specialist and do not treat them yourself.

Finally, remember to eat a protein rich snack before exercising and drink fluids containing glucose as you exercise to help maintain steady blood sugar levels during the exercise period.

***

2.

Loose Excess Weight

Losing excess weight is vital especially for those with noninsulin dependent diabetes since it can help them achieve optimum blood sugar control. This weight loss does not have to be dramatic since losing just 5% to 10% of the weight can lower blood sugar levels.

Before embarking on a weight loss plan, consult your doctor and nutritionist since your medications and diet may need to be tweaked to maintain tight blood sugar control.

***

3.

Manage Stress

Effective stress management is important for managing diabetes since when a person is under stress, the body naturally increases the amount of glucose in the bloodstream to help with the fight or flight response.

Chronic stress can therefore result in poorly controlled blood sugar levels and this can increase the risk of developing diabetic complications. Therefore, practice relaxation techniques regularly for effective stress management.

***

4.

Stop Smoking

Join a smoking cessation program and stop smoking since smoking increases the risk of diabetics developing complications like strokes, heart disease, kidney disease and erectile dysfunction.

***

5.

Get Adequate Sleep

Get 7-10 hours of sleep every night since it can help you maintain a normal body weight. This is due to the fact that the production of grehlin, an appetite stimulant, decreases during sleep while that of letpin, an appetite suppressant, increases. If you have trouble sleeping, follow these simple sleep hygiene tips:

a. Set regular bedtime and waking up times and abide by them.

b. Avoid alcohol, caffeine and nicotine intake 4-6 hours before bedtime.

c. Avoid vigorous exercises 4-6 hours before bedtime.

d. Eat a light snack before bed but avoid large meals at bedtime.

e. Eat snacks consisting of bananas, dates, milk, whole grain crackers and yogurt as these are rich in tryptophan which promotes sleep.

f. Establish a regular relaxing unwinding routine. This can include a taking a warm bath and reading a calming book such as the Bible on a kindle as you listen to soothing music.

***

6.

Foster Spiritual Health

Develop a strong spiritual relationship with God since several studies have shown that people of faith are healthier than non-believers. Other studies have also shown that prayer can reduce the symptoms of some diseases.

Having a relationship with your God can also help you cope with the stress and depression of living with a chronic condition like diabetes and deal with its complications better.

Therefore, find a Bible preaching Church and practice your faith sincerely since simply going through the motions does not confer any of the faith related health benefits.

* * * * *

6

EXERCISE PLAN

A balanced exercise plan should combine stretching, weight bearing and aerobic exercises.

If you have been leading a sedentary lifestyle, consult your doctor and nutritionist before making changes to your exercise regimen.

In addition, invest in a good pair of sports shoes that will cushion your feet and redistribute your weight evenly as you walk, jog, jump or run.

If as you exercise, you experience any of the following symptoms, stop exercising at once and consult your doctor: chest pain, pressure or tightness, unusual shortness of breath, pain in the jaw, arm, neck or shoulder, palpitations or skipped heart beats, feeling dizzy or fainting, muscle pain that is more severe than just discomfort.

1.

Stretching Exercises

Stretch for at least 10 minutes each morning and evening and in the warm up and cool down periods just before or right after your exercise sessions.

To stretch correctly you should:

1. Not hold your breath as you stretch. Breathe in and out rhythmically.

2. Never bounce into or out of your stretches. Gently move into and out of the various positions.

3. Hold the stretch position for 10 seconds and gradually increase the duration.

4. Be systematic and begin with the legs as you work your way up the body to the neck or vice versa.

5. Stop stretching if you feel any pain but continue if you experience mild discomfort.

The following is a list of exercises that you can do at home to stretch your entire body.

1. Neck Stretch - Stand with your feet shoulder width apart and your chin on your chest. Rotate your head once clockwise. Return chest to chin and rotate it counter clockwise. Do several rotations. Turn your face to the right, look as far back over your shoulder as you can. Hold for a count of 10. Repeat on opposite side.

2. Chest, Shoulder and Arm Stretch - Stand with your feet shoulder width apart and your knees slightly bent. Clasp your hands behind your back and push them back as far as you can reach. Push your chest forward as far as it can reach. Hold and return to starting position.

3. Side Stretch - Stand straight with your arms raised over your head. Tilt your body to the left side as you stretch your side muscles. Hold. Repeat on the opposite side.

4. Abs, Glutes and Quads Stretch - Stand with your feet together. Reach forward with your right arm. Lift your left leg behind you and grasp your left ankle with your left hand. Lift your left thigh as high as you can or until it is parallel to the ground. Repeat on opposite side.

5. Back Stretch - Lie on your back and pull both knees to your chest. Release them and lower your knees to the right side and then to the left side. Return knees back to chest.

6. Hamstring Stretch - Lie on your back with your legs bent and both feet flat on the floor. Straighten and raise your right leg. Gently pull your right thigh towards your body and hold for a count of 10. Repeat on the opposite side.

***

2.

Weight Bearing Exercises

To weight train or strength train correctly you should:

a) Not hold your breath or strain as you train.

b) Not exercise the same muscle groups for two consecutive days.

c) Aim for 3 sets of 10 repetitions each.

The following are exercises that you can do at home to strength train your entire body.

1. Overhead Press - (Works shoulders) Sit on a chair; hold a weight (or a full water bottle) in each hand at shoulder level with palms facing forward. Raise your arms straight up over your head. Lower them to shoulder level.

2. Biceps Curl - (Works biceps) Sit on a chair; hold a weight (or a full water bottle) in each hand palms facing forward. Bend your elbow and lift the weight towards your shoulder. Return to starting position and repeat with the other arm.

3. Triceps Dips - (Works triceps) Sit on the edge of a sturdy chair with your back and shoulders straight. Hold the edge of a chair and bend your elbows to form a right angle as you lower your butt off the seat to the floor. Straighten your arms and press back up to raise your butt back to the seat.

4. Push Ups - (Works deltoids, triceps, pectorals) Lie on floor, palms face down, elbows bent next to shoulders. Push up from floor by straightening elbows and contracting abs so that your body forms a straight line from your head to heel (beginners can rest both knees on floor) Lower yourself to floor by bending elbows. Push back up.

5. Simple Straight Crunches - (Works abs) Lie flat on your back; bend knees while keeping your feet flat on the floor. Place your hands on your thighs. Exhale and lift shoulder blades from the floor as you slide your hands up to your knees. Hold for a count of 10. Return to starting position and repeat.

6. Simple Side Crunches - (Works abs) Lie flat on your back; bend knees while keeping your feet flat on the floor. Place your hands on your right thigh. Exhale and lift shoulder blades from the floor as you slide your hands up to your right knee. Hold for a count of 10. Return to starting position and repeat. Do on opposite side.

7. Advanced Straight Crunches - (Works abs) Lie flat on your back; bend your knees until thighs are perpendicular to floor. Place arms crossed over your chest. Exhale, tighten abs and lift shoulder blades from the floor as you reach towards knees. Hold for a count of 10. Return to starting position and repeat.

8. Advanced Side Crunches - (Works abs) Lie flat on your back; bend your knees until thighs are perpendicular to floor. Place arms crossed over your chest. Exhale, tighten abs and lift shoulder blades from floor as you reach towards right knee. Hold for a count of 10. Return to starting position and repeat. Do on opposite side.

9. Leg Lifts - Lie on your back; legs straight; hands under butt. Lift legs 30 cm from the floor. Hold for a count of 10.

10. Lunge - (Works glutes, hamstrings, quadriceps) Stand with feet shoulder width apart, arms at sides. Take a large step forward with your left leg and ensure your left knee is above your left foot. Lower your body to the floor by bending the right knee until right thigh is parallel to the floor and right knee is close to the ground. Squeeze your glutes as you press back up to your starting position. Repeat on opposite side.

11. Squat - (Works your butt and thighs) Stand with your feet parallel and shoulder width apart. Stretch out your hands in front of you. Keeping your abs and butt tight, bend your knees and slowly lower yourself as though you are sitting. Ensure your knees don't extend past your toes. Hold for a count of 10. As your rise, squeeze your glutes.

12. Calf Raises - (Work your calf muscles) Stand with feet together and arms raised above your head. Lift your heels so that you are standing on the balls of your feet/toes. Stand on your toes for a count of 10.

***

3.

Aerobic Exercises

Aerobic exercises include walking, skipping a rope, jogging (on a treadmill or in the park), cycling or spinning in the gym, swimming, aerobic classes in a gym, sports like tennis and basketball as well as everyday activities like climbing stairs, housework and gardening.

Swimming is a good option especially if you are overweight or obese because it does not put excessive pressure on the joints of the lower limbs.

To reap the most benefits from your aerobic exercise sessions, you should:

1. Exercise for at least 30 min each session

2. Reach your Target Heart Rate (THR) which is calculated by

220 - your age = maximum heart rate (MHR)

MHR x 0.65 = minimum target heart rate (MinTHR)

MHR x 0.80 = maximum target heart rate (MaxTHR)

For example, if you are 40 years old, 220 - 40 years = 180 your maximum heart rate (MHR)

180 (MHR) x 0.65 = 117 your minimum target heart rate (MinTHR)

180 (MHR) x 0.80 = 144 your maximum target heart rate (MaxTHR)

Therefore, as you exercise, you should ensure that your heart rate is between 117 and 144.

To know your heart rate per minute, take your pulse on your wrist or neck for one minute.

The following is a rough guide of target heart rates for different age groups:

If you are 20 years old, your Target Heart Rate (THR) per minute should be 130 - 160

If you are 30 years old, your Target Heart Rate (THR) per minute should be 123 – 152

If you are 40 years old, your Target Heart Rate (THR) per minute should be 117 – 144

If you are 50 years old, your Target Heart Rate (THR) per minute should be 110 – 136

If you are 60 years old, your Target Heart Rate (THR) per minute should be 104 – 128

If you are 70 years old, your Target Heart Rate (THR) per minute should be 97 – 120

If you are 80 years old, your Target Heart Rate (THR) per minute should be 91 – 112

***

Exercise Plan

You can modify this plan to suit your lifestyle and level of activity.

Exercise Activity for Week 1

Day 1

Whole body stretch to warm up

30 min walk at minimum THR

Whole body stretch to cool down

Day 2

Whole body stretch to warm up

10 push ups, 10 triceps dips, 10 crunches

Whole body stretch to cool down

Day 3

Whole body stretch to warm up

30 min walk at minimum THR

Whole body stretch to cool down

Day 4

Whole body stretch to warm up

10 squats, 10 lunges, 10 calf raises, 10 crunches

Whole body stretch to cool down

Day 5

Whole body stretch to warm up

30 min walk at minimum THR

Whole body stretch to cool down

Exercise Activity for week 2

Day 1

Whole body stretch to warm up

30 min walk/ jog at medium THR

Whole body stretch to cool down

Day 2

Whole body stretch to warm up

15 push ups, 15 bicep curls, 15 triceps dips, 15 crunches

Whole body stretch to cool down

Day 3

Whole body stretch to warm up

30 min walk/ jog at medium THR

Whole body stretch to cool down

Day 4

Whole body stretch to warm up

15 squats, 15 lunges, 15 calf raises, 15 crunches

Whole body stretch to cool down

Day 5

Whole body stretch to warm up

30 min walk/ jog at medium THR

Whole body stretch to cool down

Exercise Activity for week 3

Day 1

Whole body stretch to warm up

30 min walk/run maximum THR

Whole body stretch to cool down

Day 2

Whole body stretch to warm up

20 push ups, 20 bicep curls, 20 triceps dips, 20 crunches

Whole body stretch to cool down

Day 3

Whole body stretch to warm up

30 min walk/run maximum THR

Whole body stretch to cool down

Day 4

Whole body stretch to warm up

20 squats, 20 lunges, 20 calf raises, 20 crunches

Whole body stretch to cool down

Day 5

Whole body stretch to warm up

30 min walk/run maximum THR

Whole body stretch to cool down

Exercise Activity for week 4

Day 1

Whole body stretch to warm up

30 min walk/run maximum THR

Whole body stretch to cool down

Day 2

Whole body stretch to warm up

30 push ups, 30 bicep curls, 30 triceps dips, 30 crunches

Whole body stretch to cool down

Day 3

Whole body stretch to warm up

30 min walk/run maximum THR

Whole body stretch to cool down

Day 4

Whole body stretch to warm up

30 push ups, 30 bicep curls, 30 triceps dips, 30 crunches

Whole body stretch to cool down

Day 5

Whole body stretch to warm up

30 min walk/run maximum THR

Whole body stretch to cool down

* * * * *

7

STRESS MANAGEMENT PLAN

Learning and practicing relaxation techniques is a very effective way of managing stress. These relaxation techniques include:

1.

Meditation

Meditation is another effective relaxation technique for coping with stress. To meditate, simply lie down in a quiet place and take several deep breaths. Once your body begins to feel calmer, focus on your inhalation and on the pure oxygen entering your body. As you exhale, envision you whole body relaxing. You can also meditate on Scriptures like **With God all things are possible** (Matthew 19:26) and envisioning your stressful situation resolving miraculously.

***

2.

Abdominal Breathing

Abdominal breathing or deep breathing is one fastest ways of counteracting the body's stress response. It is done by inhaling through your nose until your abdomen rises, holding your breath for a few moments and then exhaling completely through your mouth until your abdomen collapses. This cycle of filling the lungs with air, pausing and then emptying them can be repeated for 15 minutes every day.

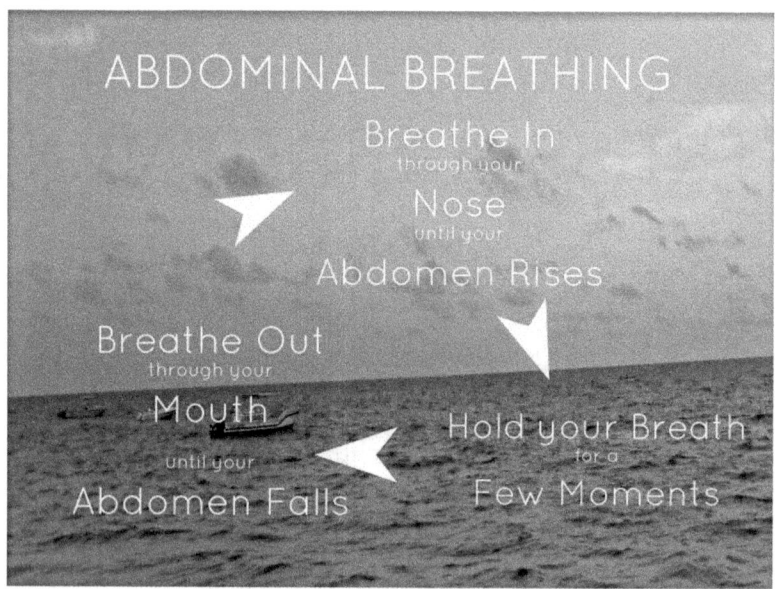

***

3.

Guided Imagery

Guided imagery is another effective relaxation technique. It involves visualizing yourself in a relaxing environment. Therefore close your eyes, take several deep breaths and use your mind's eye to see yourself relaxing on a beach or floating on a cloud or walking through a garden or whichever environment makes you feel relaxed. Use all your senses to immerse yourself in the restful environment by seeing soothing images, smelling appealing scents, hearing calming sounds, tasting and feeling your way through it. After you have enjoyed our visit, bring yourself gently back to reality.

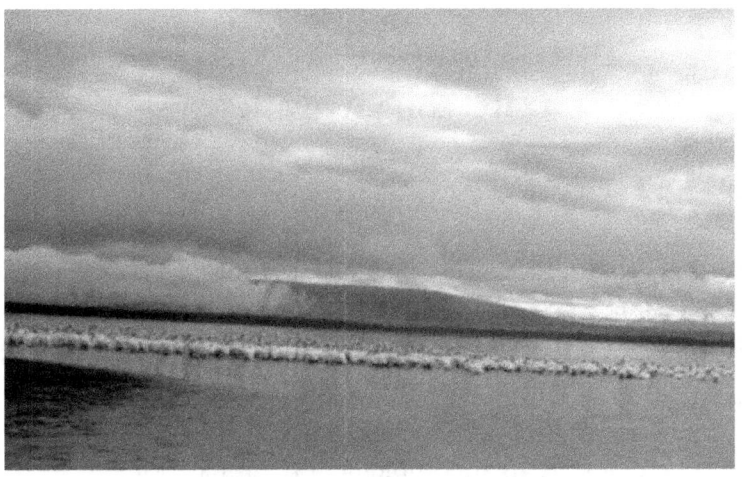

***

4.

Problem Solving Visualization

Visualization can also be used to manage stressful situations. To do this see yourself with your mind's eye in your most stressful situation and then envisioning yourself using various strategies to cope. For example you can imagine yourself dealing with a stressful boss by breathing deeply until you no longer feel distressed by their words or actions.

***

5.

Physical Exercise

When a person is stressed, they tense their muscles. Stretching exercises reduce this muscle tension and help a person feel relaxed.

Aerobic exercises help the body burn circulating stress hormones that contribute to the development of stress related illnesses.

Weight bearing exercises also aid in stress management since they demand concentration and help a person forget their problems.

Therefore engage in regular physical exercises to manage stress.

***

Relaxing Activities

Other relaxing activities that you can engage in to manage stress include:

1. Journaling since writing down uncensored feelings is a very effective method of catharsis. It is doubly effective when combined with writing lists of things you are thankful for.

2. Listening to calming music.

3. Engaging in hobbies that complement their main job

4. Helping less fortunate members of your society like visiting the sick in hospitals since this takes your mind off your problems

5. Drinking soothing herbal teas like chamomile and passionflower.

6. Eating foods which raise serotonin levels like turkey, salmon, chicken, cheese, chocolate, wholegrain bread.

7. Watching comedy since laughter relieves tension.

8. Spending time with your social support system.

***

Stress Management Plan

Stress Management Plan Week 1

Day 1

1. Abdominal breathing

2. Meditation

3. Physical Exercise

4. Watching Comedy

Day 2

1. Abdominal breathing

2. Meditation

3. Drinking herbal teas and eating serotonin rich foods

4. Watching Comedy

Day 3

1. Abdominal breathing

2. Meditation

3. Physical Exercise

4. Watching Comedy

Day 4

1. Abdominal breathing

2. Meditation

3. Drinking herbal teas and eating serotonin rich foods

4. Watching Comedy

Day 5

1. Abdominal breathing

2. Meditation

3. Physical Exercise

4. Watching Comedy

Day 6 and 7

1. Abdominal breathing 2. Meditation 3. Spending time with your social support system

Stress Management Plan Week 2

Day 1

1. Abdominal breathing

2. Guided imagery

3. Physical Exercise

4. Listening to Music

Day 2

1. Abdominal breathing

2. Guided imagery

3. Drinking herbal teas and eating serotonin rich foods

4. Listening to Music

Day 3

1. Abdominal breathing

2. Guided imagery

3. Physical Exercise

4. Listening to Music

Day 4

1. Abdominal breathing

2. Guided imagery

3. Drinking herbal teas and eating serotonin rich foods

4. Listening to Music

Day 5

1. Abdominal breathing

2. Guided imagery

3. Physical Exercise

4. Listening to Music

Day 6 and 7

1. Abdominal breathing 2. Guided imagery 3. Engaging in Complementary Hobbies

Stress Management Plan Week 3

Day 1

1. Abdominal breathing

2. Problem solving visualization

3. Physical Exercise

4. Journaling and writing gratitude lists

Day 2

1. Abdominal breathing

2. Problem solving visualization

3. Drinking herbal teas and eating serotonin rich foods

4. Journaling and writing gratitude lists

Day 3

1. Abdominal breathing

2. Problem Solving Visualization

3. Physical Exercise

4. Journaling and writing gratitude lists

Day 4

1. Abdominal breathing

2. Problem Solving Visualization

3. Drinking herbal teas and eating serotonin rich foods

4. Journaling and writing gratitude lists

Day 5

1. Abdominal breathing

2. Problem Solving Visualization

3. Physical Exercise

4. Journaling and writing gratitude lists

Day 6 and 7

1. Abdominal breathing 2. Problem Solving Visualization 3. Helping the less fortunate

Stress Management Plan Week 4

Day 1

1. Abdominal breathing

2. Meditation or Guided Imagery or Problem Solving Visualization (choose the one that has been most relaxing for you and practice it regularly)

3. Physical exercise

4. Watching Comedy or Listening to Music or Journaling and writing gratitude lists (choose the one that has been most relaxing for you and practice it regularly)

Day 2

1. Abdominal breathing

2. Meditation or Guided Imagery or Problem Solving Visualization (choose the one that has been most relaxing for you and practice it regularly)

3. Drinking herbal teas and eating serotonin rich foods

4. Watching Comedy or Listening to Music or Journaling and writing gratitude lists (choose the one that has been most relaxing for you and practice it regularly)

Day 3

1. Abdominal breathing

2. Meditation or Guided Imagery or Problem Solving Visualization (choose the one that has been most relaxing for you and practice it regularly)

3. Physical exercise

4. Watching Comedy or Listening to Music or Journaling and writing gratitude lists (choose the one that has been most relaxing for you and practice it regularly)

Day 4

1. Abdominal breathing

2. Meditation or Guided Imagery or Problem Solving Visualization (choose the one that has been most relaxing for you and practice it regularly)

3. Drinking herbal teas and eating serotonin rich foods

4. Watching Comedy or Listening to Music or Journaling and writing gratitude lists (choose the one that has been most relaxing for you and practice it regularly)

Day 5

1. Abdominal breathing

2. Meditation or Guided Imagery or Problem Solving Visualization (choose the one that has been most relaxing for you and practice it regularly)

3. Physical exercise

4. Watching Comedy or Listening to Music or Journaling and writing gratitude lists (choose the one that has been most relaxing for you and practice it regularly)

Day 6 and 7

1. Abdominal breathing

2. Meditation or Guided Imagery or Problem Solving Visualization (choose the one that has been most relaxing for you and practice it regularly)

3. Spending time with your social support system or Engaging in complementary hobbies or Helping the less fortunate (choose the one that has been most relaxing for you and practice it regularly)

###

ABOUT THE AUTHOR

Dr. Miriam Kinai is a medical doctor and freelance health writer/blogger.

You can visit her blog at http://www.MyBlogBookClub.com or follow her on twitter at http://twitter.com/AlmasiHealth

Email enquiries to almasihealthcare@yahoo.com with BOOKS as your subject.

HERBS AND SPICES FOR THE COOK, HEALER AND BEAUTICIAN

Herbs and Spices for the Cook, Healer and Beautician uses color pictures and clear explanations to teach you about more than 70 healing herbs and spices.

You will learn about their:

* Therapeutic (healing) uses

* Drug interactions

* Contraindications (when not to use them)

* Cooking tips

* Beauty tips

*****

INTERNATIONAL GOURMET HERB AND SPICE BLENDS

International Gourmet Herb and Spice Blends teaches you how to prepare exotic herb and spice blends from around the world. You will discover the recipes for:

* Barbecue Rub, Cajun, Apple Pie and Pumpkin Pie Spice Mixes from America

* Pudding Spice Mix from Britain

* 5 Spice Mix from China

* Berbere Spice Mix from Ethiopia

* Curry Powder and Garam Masala from India

* Bouquet Garni, Herbs de Provence and Quatre Epices from France

* Herb Mix from Italy

* Jerk Seasoning from Jamaica

* Shichimi Togarashi from Japan

* Pilau Spice Blend from Kenya

* Chili Powder from Mexico

* Baharat Spice Blend from the Middle East

* Ras El Hanout from Morocco

*****

THE QUICK GOURMET CHEF

The Quick Gourmet is an essential culinary skills cookbook which teaches how to make simple, divine dishes.

You will learn how to make:

* Hot Chocolate Mixes and Drinks

* Hot Chai Tea Mixes and Drinks

* Hot Coffee Mixes and Drinks

* Sensational Smoothies

* Non-Dairy Smoothies

* Chocolate Covered Strawberries

* Chocolate Truffles

* Healthy Chicken Salads

* Healthy Tuna Salads

* Savory Salsas

* Herb Butter

* Cheese Dips and Sauces

* Gourmet Sandwiches

* Perfect Hard Boiled Eggs

* A Cheese Board

* Natural Food Color

*****

HOW TO STYLE AND PHOTOGRAPH FOOD

Regardless of whether you are an aspiring food blogger or you want to make money online selling stock photos, How To Style and Photograph Food, uses color pictures and clear explanations to teach you the food photography tips that can help you improve your digital camera photography skills so that you can begin photographing food like a pro.

You will learn:

* The equipment that you need

* How to set up the lighting

* How to prepare the stage

* How to style the food

* How to shoot the food

*****

HOW TO MAKE NATURAL SKIN CARE PRODUCTS VOLUME 1

How To Make Natural Skin Care Products Volume 1 by Dr Miriam Kinai is filled with recipes for making organic bath and body products for normal, sensitive, oily and dry skin types as well as therapeutic products to manage mature skin, prematurely aging skin, cellulite, eczema, psoriasis, ringworms, dandruff, thinning hair, menopausal symptoms, pre-menstrual tension (PMS), painful periods, arthritis, stress, sadness or depression, mental exhaustion and insomnia.

This book also teaches you the best vegetable oils, essential oils, natural butters and herbs to use when making products for different skin types physical conditions. You will learn how to make:

* Bath bombs

* Bath melts

* Bath salts

* Bath teas

* Body butters

* Body lotions

* Body scrubs

* Healing balms and body creams

* Herb infused oils

* Natural soap

How to Make Natural Skin Care Products Volume 1 will leave you with a clear understanding of how to make bath and beauty products to use in your home or to give as gifts or to sell and make money.

*****

ORGANIC SKIN CARE PRODUCT INGREDIENTS

Organic Skin Care Product Ingredients teaches you about the different natural substances that can be used to create natural bath and beauty products to use in your home or to give as gifts to your loved ones or to sell and make money.

You will learn about:

* Natural butters

* Natural clays

* Natural colorants

* Natural exfoliants

* Natural fragrances

* Natural oils

* Natural preservatives

*****

THE ESSENTIALS OF AROMATHERAPY ESSENTIAL OILS

The Essentials of Aromatherapy Essential Oils by Dr Miriam Kinai teaches you how to use aromatherapy oils to improve your physical, mental and emotional well being.

The author's experience as a medical doctor and clinical aromatherapy practitioner have enabled her to write a highly informative guide for those who want to utilize the healing benefits of these natural plant essences.

You will discover:

* The safety information and therapeutic uses of 18 essential oils

* How to blend essential oils

* The characteristics and uses of 14 carrier oils

* How to Dilute Essential Oils with Carrier Oils

* How to Use Essential Oils

* Cautionary Measures when using Essential Oils

* Numerous Essential Oil Recipes for bath products as well as skin care and hair care products

The Essentials of Aromatherapy Essential Oils will leave you with a clear understanding of how you can safely use aromatherapy essential oils to heal yourself naturally.

*****

CARRIER OILS GUIDE

Carrier Oils Guide teaches you the characteristics, health benefits and uses of commonly used carrier oils. You will learn about:

* Apricot Kernel Oil

* Avocado Oil

* Borage Seed Oil

* Calendula Oil

* Carrot Seed Oil

* Castor Oil

* Evening Primrose Oil

* Fractionated Coconut Oil

* Jojoba

* Olive Oil

* Rosehip Oil

* Sunflower Oil

* Sweet Almond Oil

* Virgin Coconut Oil

* Useful formulas for Diluting Essential Oils with Carrier Oils

*****

MEDICAL AROMATHERAPY FOR HEALTH PROFESSIONALS

Medical Aromatherapy for Healthcare Professionals by Dr Miriam Kinai teaches you how to use essential oils to treat physical diseases and emotional disorders.

The author's experience as a medical doctor and clinical aromatherapy practitioner have enabled her to write a highly informative guide for those who want to utilize the healing benefits of these natural plant essences.

You will discover how to use essential oils to:

* Treat skin diseases like acne, eczema and psoriasis

* Treat other physical diseases like high blood pressure, arthritis, coughs and colds

* Manage mental and emotional conditions like anxiety, depression, anger and stress

* Relieve the symptoms of menopause and premenstrual tension

* Lessen insomnia and impotence

Medical Aromatherapy for Healthcare Professionals is therefore an essential resource for holistic healthcare practitioners like massage therapists, naturopaths and herbalists.

It is also a useful resource for conventional medicine healthcare providers like physicians and nurses who want to begin practicing integrative medicine and for patients who want to improve their health naturally by using aromatherapy oils.

*****

AROMATHERAPY COURSE

Aromatherapy Course by Dr Miriam Kinai tutors you on how to use essential oils to improve your physical, mental and emotional well being.

The author's experience as a medical doctor and clinical aromatherapy practitioner have enabled her to create a highly informative course on how to use these natural plant essences.

You will learn:

* The safety information and therapeutic uses of essential oils like clary sage, eucalyptus, geranium, grapefruit, lavender, lemon, lemongrass, marjoram, orange (sweet), patchouli, peppermint, Roman chamomile, rose, rosemary, sandalwood, spearmint, tea tree and ylang ylang.

* The safety information and therapeutic uses of carrier oils like apricot kernel oil, avocado oil, borage seed oil, calendula oil, carrot seed oil, castor oil, evening primrose oil, fractionated coconut oil, jojoba, olive oil, rosehip oil, sunflower oil, sweet almond oil and virgin coconut oil.

* How to blend essential oils

* How to dilute essential oils with carrier oils

* How to administer essential oils

* How to make natural healing products from numerous aromatherapy recipes

* How to utilize the healing benefits of essentials oils even if you do not have prior training in aromatherapy

The Aromatherapy Course will leave you with a clear understanding of how you can heal yourself and your family naturally by using essentials oils on your body and in your home.

*****

DEALING WITH DEPRESSION NATURALLY

Dealing with Depression Naturally presents a holistic approach to managing depression with natural antidepressants. You will learn how to treat depression with:

* Aromatherapy

* Art therapy

* Christian Biblical principles

* Chromotherapy

* Diet therapy

* Eco-therapy

* Herbal therapy

* Home decor therapy

* Music therapy

* Phototherapy

* Exercise therapy

* Self-Psychotherapy

* Social therapy

* Talk therapy

* Vitamin therapy

* Writing therapy

*****

CHRISTIAN LIFE COACHING HANDBOOK

Christian Life Coaching Handbook offers a Biblical approach to managing different aspects of life.

You will learn:

* Christian anger management

* Christian conflict resolution

* Christian depression treatment

* Christian goal setting

* Christian marital stress management

* Christian stress management

* How to assert yourself

* How to defeat fear

* How to love yourself

* How to overcome shyness

* How to resist temptation

* How to stop being a people pleaser

*****

CHRISTIAN PERSONAL FINANCE

Christian Personal Finance teaches Biblical principles of money management.

You will learn:

* Christian financial stress management from people who were dealing with money stress like the Acts 3 beggar or credit issues like the widow in second Kings.

* Biblical prosperity principles from wealthy men and women of God like Isaac and the Proverbs 31 woman.

* Bible verses to use as spiritual warfare prayers and as Christian finance affirmations and Christian money meditations.

*****

ANTHOLOGY OF CHRISTIAN BIBLE SERMONS

Anthology of Christian Bible Sermons is a compilation of more than 20 Biblical rhema teachings which include:

* A New Christmas Message

* A New Easter Message

* Are You A Flamboyant Fig Tree Christian?

* Biblical Lessons for Purim from Queen Esther

* Can God Help Me If I Am Surrounded By Enemies?

* How Badly Do You Really Want It?

* Seed Words And The Powerful Tongue

* Spiritual AIDS

* The Three Levels Of Getting Lost

* Why Does God Allow Suffering?

* Your Life Is Your Ministry And Your Storm Is Your Message

* A Perfect God, Imperfect People, and Perfect Plans

* We Are Not Ignorant of His Devices

* How to Prepare for a Dangerous Journey

* Yes, God Can

* How to Serve the Body of Christ

* Conduits of God

* Go Back? Stand Still? Move Forward? Drown?

*****

CHRISTIAN SPIRITUAL WARFARE

Christian Spiritual Warfare teaches you the awesome Bible verses you can use as spiritual warfare prayers, Christian affirmations and in your Christian meditation sessions as you fight your spiritual battles.

You will learn how to fight for the following with Bible verses:

* Marriage * Children * Health

* Christian Faith * Christian Ministry

* Country

* Finances * Job * Business

* Peace of Mind * Restoration * Self Esteem * Self Love

You will also learn how to fight against the following with Bible verses:

* Addiction * Temptation

* Being Single * Infertility

* Opposition * Oppression

* Worry * Fear

* Feelings of Condemnation * Confusion

* Danger * Death * Despair * Discouragement

* Impatience * Insomnia * Laziness * Loneliness

* Poverty * Pride * Sadness

* Vengeance * Weakness

* A Foul Mouth * Lying

*****

DARK SKIN DERMATOLOGY COLOR ATLAS

Dark Skin Dermatology Color Atlas is filled with clear explanations and color photos of skin, hair, and nail diseases affecting people with skin of color or Fitzpatrick skin types IV, V, and VI.

Topics covered include Acne Vulgaris, Alopecia Areata, Anal Warts, Angioedema, Aphthous Ulcers, Atopic Dermatitis, Blastomycosis, Blister Beetle Dermatitis or Nairobi Fly Dermatitis, Cellulitis, Chronic Ulcers, Confetti Hypopigmentation, Cutaneous T Cell Lymphoma, Cutaneous Tuberculosis, Dermatitis Artefacta, Erythema Nodosum,

Exfoliative Erythroderma, Gianotti Crosti Syndrome, Hand Dermatitis, Hemangioma, Herpes Zoster, Ichthyosis, Ingrown Toenails, Irritant Contact Dermatitis, Kaposi Sarcoma, Keloids, Keratoderma Blenorrhagica, Klippel Trenaunay Weber Syndrome, Leishmaniasis, Leprosy, Leukonychia, Lichen Nitidus, Lichen Planus,

Lichenoid Drug Eruption, Linear Epidermal Nevus, Linear IgA Dermatosis (LAD), Lipodermatosclerosis, Lymphangioma Circumscriptum, Miliaria, Molluscum Contagiosum, Neurofibromatosis, Nickel Dermatitis, Onychomadesis, Onychomycosis, Palmoplantar Eccrine Hidradenitis, Papular Pruritic Eruption (PPE), Paronychia, Pellagra, Pemphigus Foliaceous,

Pemphigus Vulgaris, Piebaldism, Pityriasis Rosea, Pityriasis Rubra Pilaris, Plantar Hyperkeratosis, Plantar Warts, Poikiloderma, Postinflammatory Hyperpigmentation and Hypopigmentation, Post Topical Steroids Hypopigmentation, Psoriasis, Pyogenic Granuloma or Lobular Capillary Hemangioma, Scabies, Seborrheic Dermatitis, Steven Johnson Syndrome (SJS) and Toxic Epidermal Necrolysis (TEN),

Sunburn, Systemic Sclerosis, Tinea Capitis, Tinea Pedis, Tinea Versicolor, Traction Alopecia, Urticaria, Vasculitis, Vitiligo, and Xanthelasma.

*****